Seven Secrets of a Healthy and Attractive Mouth

A beautiful smile is a great asset, develop yours

Dr. Ola Lawson

Bloomington, IN

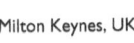

authorHOUSE®

Milton Keynes, UK

AuthorHouse™
1663 Liberty Drive, Suite 200
Bloomington, IN 47403
www.authorhouse.com
Phone: 1-800-839-8640

AuthorHouse™ UK Ltd.
500 Avebury Boulevard
Central Milton Keynes, MK9 2BE
www.authorhouse.co.uk
Phone: 08001974150

This book is not meant to be a substitute for personal dental advice but as a supplement for the person who desires to develop and maintain a healthy and attractive mouth.

First published by AuthorHouse 9/2/2007

ISBN: 978-1-4343-1718-6 (e)
ISBN: 978-1-4259-9475-4 (sc)

Printed in the United States of America
Bloomington, Indiana

This book is printed on acid-free paper.

Contents

INTRODUCTION

Hello!

I'm delighted you've picked up this book. I will be taking you on an adventure to discover the secrets behind having a mouth that anyone would envy. I have learned these secrets in the course of many years of dental practice.

You will agree with me that a good smile is a great asset. Your mouth can either attract people or make them find the slightest excuse to turn away. It is the gateway that controls so much in our lives – what goes in, as well as what comes out by way of words.

Your lipstick, even though nice and attractive, may lose its appeal if what lies behind it needs attention. An expensive well-cut suit with a cute tie does not display its true value if the smile above it reminds you of 'Jaws'. You may get away talking with your date on the phone, but what happens when you meet face to face?

You may still be wondering why I've decided to write a book on the mouth. Wait for a moment and consider this statement:

Out of all the things you wear, your expression, to

which your mouth contributes a great deal, is the greatest.

When looked after, the mouth can be a source of pleasure; but it can also cause a lot of discomfort if care is not taken.

I'm sure, by now, you're eager to accompany me on this rewarding adventure. No matter what condition your mouth is in, you can bring it to a state of health.

It's your choice.

SECRET 1: HAVE A GOOD KNOWLEDGE OF YOUR MOUTH

Every instruction manual begins by showing you a labelled picture of whatever it is you've bought. It does this in order to give you an idea of the different parts to enable you to follow the operating instructions. In the same way a good driving instructor will show his student all the different parts of a car, especially the brakes, before allowing him or her to drive.

In this chapter I will be discussing the different parts of the mouth. The word mouth means opening or entrance. Many people think of their teeth as the only part of the mouth. Teeth might be the most obvious, but they are certainly not the only part. The mouth is a collection of different parts with different functions, all working together in harmony. It is a very sensitive part of the body that we often take for granted until something goes wrong.

Starting from the outside, the mouth consists of:

LIPS: These obviously consist of two parts, the upper and the lower lip, and come in different shapes and sizes. In addition to other functions, they serve as the gate to the inner part of the mouth.

GUMS: These cover the bones and the necks of the teeth, and are also called *gingivae.*

TONGUE: This is a strong but sensitive muscular structure that helps control the movement of food around the mouth, and also, as you know, plays an important role in talking.

TEETH: As I said before, especially when they are gleaming white, these are the most obvious part of the mouth. They are used for breaking down food so that it can be easily swallowed. There are four different kinds: incisors, canines, premolars and molars. Each is designed for a different function.

TONSILS: These are in the throat behind the mouth, and are part of the body's immune or defence system.

I will also mention briefly the contents of the mouth:

SALIVA: This is the mouth's lubricant. It is produced by the salivary glands located in different parts of the mouth, and keeps the mouth moist and the different parts working effectively together. It also makes swallowing easy. In fact, through the action of enzymes contained in the saliva, the process of digestion begins in the mouth. Saliva also helps to prevent infection in the mouth.

BACTERIA: Although we cannot see them, these are also present in the mouth and, given the opportunity, will certainly make their presence known. Accumulation of these bacteria can be seen as a sticky, whitish film which forms on your teeth daily and can be scrapped off their surfaces. This is called plaque, and is your number one enemy. It binds to teeth, allowing the acids produced by the bacteria to damage them. Plaque after a while becomes mineralised to form tartar. This is not easily removed. A good knowedge of how to deal with plaque will give you an advantage in the quest for an excellent mouth.

KEY POINTS

- *The mouth is a collection of different parts with different functions, all working in harmony.*
- *Plaque is your number one enemy. A good knowledge of how to deal with it will give you an advantage in the quest for an excellent mouth.*

SECRET 2: KNOW THE FUNCTIONS OF YOUR MOUTH

I went to visit my Aunty who I had not seen in a long time. After we got talking she asked her little daughter to get me a can of coke from the refrigerator. Wondering why she did not return with it, she went into the kitchen, only to find her trying to warm it up in the microwave! She obviously did not realise why the can of coke was kept in the refrigerator. When the function of something is not known, abuse is inevitable. However, a good knowledge of its functions enables us to appreciate its value and to regard it in a different way.

We will now quickly go through the different functions of the mouth. As I said in the previous chapter, the different parts of the mouth work together to produce various results.

EXPRESSION: The mouth plays an important part in facial expression, such as smiling, laughing and frowning. These expressions help in our communication with one another.

SPEECH: This is one of the main functions of the mouth. It is carried out by the tongue, lips and teeth working in harmony with the vocal cords. Defects in these parts can affect speech.

TASTING: This function is carried out by taste buds found on the tongue. They give us the sense by which we can tell the flavour of food and drink.

AFFECTION: Kissing. The mouth, probably because of its sensitive nature, is used in sharing affection.

EATING: This is probably the most obvious function. The mouth is designed specifically for eating different kinds of food.

Other functions of the mouth range from blowing up a balloon to screaming, sighing, yawning and whistling; and there are many others besides. The mouth has also the capacity to adapt, as seen in some disabled people who use their mouths to paint, write and do other things.

KEY POINTS

- *When the funtions of something is not known,abuse is inevitable*
- *A good knowledge of the mouth enables us to appreciate its value, and regard it in a different way.*

SECRET 3: BE AWARE OF CHANGES IN YOUR MOUTH

THE GOOD, THE BAD AND THE UGLY

This has nothing to do with the movie. Our title points to the fact that we need to know the signs that indicate changes in our mouths. At this stage, may I suggest that it is worth having any changes you observe checked out by your dentist.

THE GOOD
A pain free mouth is not necessarily a healthy mouth. It is possible for a lot to be going on without our noticing it for some time. A healthy mouth is one that maintains its normal structure, function and colour, and is regularly certified by a dentist as being so. It is important therefore that we know how a normal mouth should look and feel, so that any change from this condition can easily be spotted and reported. A good way of checking

is to look in the mirror regularly. This can be done quite easily when brushing.

THE BAD
Our mouth consists of different parts each of which can undergo changes. We will be looking at some of these changes here.

The gums: The most common cause of tooth loss in adults is gum disease.
Many people mistakenly think that the first sign of a diseased mouth is pain. This is not true. Changes can occur without our experiencing any discomfort, and gum disease is one of them. It begins usually unobserved and progresses painlessly, producing few outward signs. It is caused by the bacteria found in plaque (the whitish film we can scrape off our teeth) especially in the area where the teeth meet the gums. Getting rid of this plaque therefore is the fundamental way of dealing with gum disease. I will not go into too much detail, but to identify a few of the signs will be helpful. Inflamed (red or swollen) gums, bleeding from the gums(especially after brushing), receding gums, persistent bad breath, a bad taste in the mouth and wobbly teeth may all indicate gum disease which, if left untreated, may lead to losing teeth.

The teeth: Teeth generally need attention when they have a cavity – that is, a hole. Cavities are caused by the decay that results when the tooth's structure is softened by acid. Acid? Well, the real culprit is again the plaque that I referred to earlier. When bacteria in the plaque feed on sugar or tiny left-over food particles in the mouth they produce an acid which dissolves the teeth, forming a cavity or hole. The early stages of tooth decay may not be easy for you to detect, but your dentist will find them. Cavities generally get bigger and can cause toothache. At this stage, even if the outward sign does not get you to the dentist, the pain surely will.

Bad breath: Halitosis is the technical name given to bad breath. It is usually a sign that something is going on in your mouth, and the best way to tackle the problem is to go to the root of it. Many people mask their bad breath by chewing sugar-free gum. This produces only a temporary effect while the source may actually be getting worse. I always wondered why babies never seem to have bad breath until I took the time to examine the difference between an adult's and a baby's mouth. The reason had been obvious all along. They don't have teeth and we do. Even when they start growing teeth, these are usually well spaced out, which prevents food getting trapped between them. In dealing with bad breath therefore one of the main steps is to get rid of food particles stuck between your teeth. Have you ever tried smelling a piece of meat that has been stuck between your teeth for more than a day? You will be surprised at the effect it has, no matter how tiny it is. Now stretch your imagination further and picture a mouth with a bit of meat here, a bit of broccoli there, and a tiny piece of a pea right at the back between the back teeth. When such a mouth opens it will mimic a nuclear explosion. You may be wondering whether people with mouths like that brush them at all. Well, most people do, but tooth brushing on its own will not remove food stuck between your teeth. You will need to discover the areas in your mouth which are prone to harbouring food (the tongue can be very useful in doing this) and then remove it by flossing or using an interdental brush. I'll speak more about this later. It is also important to note that it is not only food that gets stuck in between teeth. Plaque does so as well, and needs to be removed.

Plaque and tartar themselves, if allowed to form in areas that can easily be cleaned, can also cause bad breath. This is usually the result of a poor brushing technique.

Another cause of bad breath is tooth decay. You cannot underestimate the effect of this, especially when the decay has spread to such an extent that the tooth itself has died.

A certain percentage of bad breath also comes from foul smelling gases produced by bacteria on the surface of the tongue. Cleaning your tongue, especially the back, may significantly reduce this.

Since the mouth is linked to other parts of the body, bad breath could also originate from problems in the stomach or adjacent regions. In such a case you should consult your doctor.

THE UGLY

I have decided to use the term "ugly" for changes that need urgent attention. It is not a pleasant word, but these changes are not pleasant either – they may develop into mouth cancer. They can affect any part of the mouth, appearing at first as an either ulcer, which though painless, does not heal normally, or as a white or red patch. If you notice an ulcer or patch that does not clear up within three weeks, please see your dentist as soon as possible.

To conclude this chapter I would repeat my advice to report any change you are not sure about to your dentist immediately.

KEY POINTS

- *A pain free mouth is not necessarily a healthy mouth.*
- *The most common cause of tooth loss in adults is gum disease.*
- *If you notice an ulcer or patch that does not clear up within three weeks, please see your dentist as soon as possible.*

SECRET 4: KNOW WHAT TO AVOID

Two friends were on their way to watch a movie. Realising that they had quite a bit of time to spare, one suggested that they should stop off at his grandma's on their way. While he chatted away with her, his friend sat at the dining table looking around for something to pass the time. Eventually he found a bowl of nuts and started to toss them into his mouth one after the other, hoping that his friend would finish soon. When they were ready to go, he noticed that his friend's grandma had no teeth. Concerned, he politely asked her what had happened to them, and how she managed to eat without them. She replied, "I dropped my teeth off for repair the other day and haven't had them back yet. I haven't been able to eat without them. I've just been able to survive by sucking chocolates and leaving the nuts out." She then proceeded to the table to show them the nuts she had been collecting, but they were all gone.

There are some things we must just learn to avoid, and I will be discussing them in this chapter.

Number one is undoubtedly smoking. I'm sorry to start off with you! Apart from its detrimental effect on the body in general, the effect of smoking on the mouth is quite destructive. Smoking reduces the oxygen in the blood stream, it also reduces the response of the body in fighting infection, thereby affecting the ability of the mouth's tissues to heal. The gums especially are affected, and this, coupled with plaque, leads to gum disease, which can progress rapidly in some cases. This aside, a large percentage of mouth cancer is linked to tobacco smoking. Some ethnic groups also chew tobacco, betel quid, pan and guttcha, and this is a recipe for disaster. Many cases of cancer have been linked to them. While still on the subject, it is worth noting that tobacco and alcohol when consumed together increase the risk of mouth cancer; also that over-exposure to sunlight carries the risk of cancer affecting the lips, and should be avoided.

Choosing to give up smoking can be one of the most important and rewarding decisions you will ever make.
Your dentist will refer you to a stop-smoking centre where you can receive advice, help and support.

Next on our list is regular consumption of sugar or sugary foods. As we said earlier, the acids produced through the action of bacteria on the sugar cause tooth decay. This means that reducing the sugar level in your mouth can effectively reduce tooth decay. If you must eat such food, I advise you to eat them at a particular time rather than spread them throughout the day. Simply put, it is better to eat a large amount of sugary food at one sitting than small amounts every hour or so, which will provide a constant supply of sugar for the bacteria to act on. In the same way, giving babies dummies soaked in honey or putting them to sleep with bottles containing sugary drinks will only cause their teeth to decay.

I know you may enjoy your fizzy drinks, but too much can wear your teeth, especially if you tend to hold them in your mouth.
Tooth wear can also be caused by repeatedly biting into fruits like apples, oranges and other citrus fruit. These contain acids that can wear down your teeth over a period of time. Of course fruits are good for us, and we should eat them, but avoid biting into them regularly. Slicing them up may be an alternative.

Another important cause of tooth wear, which can be serious, is overzealous brushing of the teeth. By this I mean brushing too hard, applying excessive force. People do this, often with good intentions, to keep their mouth really clean. After a while, however, they start complaining of sensitivity. I often tell my patients to brush, not scrub. It's not how hard you brush but how effectively.

Grinding the teeth can also cause wear which may eventually lead to the teeth being disfigured. If you notice you have such a problem, it might be a good idea to mention this to your dentist. Some people also suffer from conditions such as bulimia, that bring about reflux of the stomach content into the mouth. This contains acid and will also cause tooth wear. It is advisable to have such conditions checked.

The reason teeth should be protected from these different causes of wear is that they gradually lose their normal structure, which can eventually affect appearance.

In a bid to protect their children's teeth from decay, some parents give them regular fluoride supplements. Fluoride does indeed give protection from dental decay, but excessive intake should be avoided as it can actually damage the teeth. This is why it is advised that children use only a pea-sized portion of toothpaste when brushing, and should be encouraged to spit it out rather than swallow it.

For denture wearers, it is good practice not to keep dentures in the mouth all the time. They should be taken out at night and properly stored. This gives the mouth good breathing space to recover.

KEY POINTS

- *Tobacco and alcohol when consumed together increases the risk of mouth cancer.*
- *Reducing the sugar level in your mouth can effectively reduce tooth decay*
- *Teeth should be protected from different causes of wear.*

SECRET 5: CULTIVATE A HEALTHY EATING HABIT

Having dwelled on the negative in the last chapter, I will now allow in a breath of fresh air by considering some positive things as well. Since the most important thing that goes into our mouth is food, we will be focusing in this section on good diet.

I was watching a documentary on the eating habits of teenagers. One particular boy was asked whether he ate fruit at all. He answered, "Yes, apple pies." I am not a dietician but I do believe in moderation. Like any other part of the body, the mouth requires a well balanced diet providing all the necessary nutrients in order to maintain a healthy state.

Foods that are fibrous, like some cereals and fruits, provide mechanical cleansing while eating. Other foods, like cheese, cause more saliva to be produced which in turn provides protection and lubrication to the mouth.

A diet rich in fruit and vegetables is also advisable as it helps to protect against cancer and other diseases.

Children should be encouraged to have foods that are rich in calcium, like milk and yoghurt, as these help in the development of their teeth.

There are many diet plans out there. You have to choose the one that suits you best. However, in my opinion, moderation, a balanced diet and regular exercise will do you a lot of good.

KEY POINT

- *Moderation, a balanced diet and regular excercise will do you a lot of good.*

SECRET 6: VISIT YOUR DENTIST REGULARLY

A patient once said to a young dentist, "I'm very nervous, you know. This is my first extraction." The dentist replied, "Don't worry, this is my first extraction too!" Another patient asked his dentist to make his smile better. After several hours in the surgery he checked his teeth in the mirror and was delighted. "I'm very pleased," he told the dentist. He proceeded to the reception desk to pay for his treatment. On seeing the bill, all the veneers, crowns and fillings fell out.

There are many reasons why people don't like dentists. Often my patients say, "Oh, it's nothing personal, but I just don't like dentists." We could list so many reasons for this attitude, from previous bad experiences to paying the bill. However, in this chapter I should like to highlight the importance of the professional touch in the care of your mouth.

Firstly, the dentist is bound by oath to do whatever is best for you. I always tell my patients to feel free to ask me anything about their mouth, as it is part of my duty to advise them. The dentist is professionally trained to identify changes you might not be aware of and to advise you appropriately about treating your condition. This is the essential value of having a regular check up. Depending on the condition of your mouth, you should have one at least once a year. Your dentist will however advise you accordingly.

In certain circumstances, when your dentist cannot carry out a treatment, he will refer you for a specialist opinion and treatment. Some practices have hygienists who are trained to clean your mouth and to give you advice on the correct techniques of mouth care.

The dentist is not therefore someone who sits with a drill and can't wait to inflict pain on you. He has a professional obligation to care for you.

There are various treatments your dentist may offer, depending on what you present with. Most will draw up a treatment plan and assess what time is required to carry out each treatment. You will then be given an appointment. Some treatment may require more than one visit.

I shall now review some of the treatments dentists provide.

FILLINGS
If your dentist discovers a cavity caused by decay, you may require a filling to stop it progressing. He will use a high-speed drill to remove the decayed part and fill the resulting hole. This can be done with various materials: amalgam, which is silver in colour; composites, which are white but comes in different shades to match your teeth. Other materials are gold and porcelain.

ROOT CANAL THERAPY
Most patients go silent when you mention this treatment. It may sound alarming, but it means simply cleaning out an infected tooth, including the roots. The treatment is needed when a cavity has been left for a while, resulting in infection of the nerves and blood vessels in the tooth. At this stage, you may or may not be in pain. The treatment allows you to keep the tooth rather than have it out. It usually requires more than one visit to the dentist, who will use special files to clean the infected tooth, thereby making it sterile. The tooth is filled afterwards and may need a crown to protect it.

CROWNS
A crown is usually needed when you've lost a large part of your tooth as a result of either decay

or injury. It helps to protect the remaining tooth stucture. Providing a crown normally takes two visits. Your dentist will first shape the tooth in a special way to receive the the crown or cap. He will take an impression of your teeth and place a temporary covering on the tooth being treated. On the second visit he will fit the crown. Crowns can be made of different materials, such as gold or porcelain. Most people prefer porcelain as it can be made to match the shade of your teeth.

EXTRACTION
I really do not like the word 'impossible', but I have to admit that a time comes when it is impossible to save a tooth. Your dentist will advise you to have such a tooth extracted or removed. In a different case, if the mouth is crowded, healthy teeth may need to be removed to make room to straighten those that remain. Extraction of a tooth involves using forceps pushed down on the root surfaces. Sometimes the dentist may need to cut your gums and remove some bone to get the whole tooth out.

DENTURES
After the removal of a tooth or teeth, personal appearance and such functions as eating and speech may be affected. This calls for the replacement of the missing teeth. One method is to provide dentures, which are artificial teeth made of acrylic (plastic), metal or a mixture of

both.They are removable and need cleaning regularly. It usually takes about four to five visits to the dentist to have them made. You will need patience and perseverance to get used to them. People without any teeth can also have dentures made for them. I have made quite a few, and it's still a wonder what some people are able to do with them.

BRIDGES
Bridgework is another way of replacing missing teeth, but unlike dentures a bridge is fixed. Your dentist will assess your mouth to find out whether it is a suitable option. Bridgework involves making crowns on the tooth or teeth adjacent to the gap left by the missing tooth and attaching the replacement tooth to them. There are different types of bridges. Your dentist will normally advise you about this.

IMPLANTS
Implanting involves placing a metal tube into the bone, which is then allowed to grow around the metal making it very firm. A crown is then constucted to fit the tube. This is a highly specialised technique and your dentist, if not trained, will refer you to have it done.It is not a cheap option of replacing missing teeth.

ORTHODONTIC TREATMENT

This treatment involves straightening teeth that are crowded or are in a wrong position. It is usually carried out in children to improve the function of the mouth, or appearance. Adults may also benefit. Straightening the teeth is achieved with the use of braces, which may be fixed or removable.

Treatment may in some cases last for several months, and it is important that good oral hygiene is maintained throughout the course of treatment. Your dentist will normally refer you to an Orthodontist – the specialist who provides this treatment.

VENEERS

These are used to improve appearance. They are very thin restorations placed on the front surface of teeth and are less destructive than crowns.

BLEACHING

This is also used to improve appearance. It involves using bleaching agents to make the shade of your teeth lighter.There are regulations guiding the use of these agents. It is safer to have your treatment done by your dentist.

SCALE AND POLISH

This is simply cleaning your teeth professionally. It helps remove plaque and tatar that has built up around the teeth, and if these are minimal, it is usually a simple clean. However, if some form of gum disease has developed cleaning may extend to the root surfaces. Some dentists carry out this treatment themselves while others have hygienists who are also qualified to do so.

FISSURE SEALANTS

This treatment involves the application of a protective coating to the biting surface of permanent teeth in children, and is useful when there is significant decay in their baby teeth. The procedure needs to be carried out before decay starts on the permanent tooth surface. Again, some dentists do it themselves, others have their hygienist do it. An injection is not required and most children are quite happy to have the treatment.

PAIN CONTROL

It would be unfair to discuss all these treatments without mentioning that your dentist will offer you an injection to make them pain free. The needles used are very fine and most patients cope well with them. To make the process comfortable a gel may be applied to your gums prior to the injection. If you are very nervous your dentist will discuss with you other options of pain control.

KEY POINTS

- *The dentist has a professional obligation to care for you.*
- *Your dentist is professionally trained to identify changes you might not be aware of and to advise you appropriately about treating your condition.*

SECRET 7: TAKE CARE OF YOUR MOUTH THE RIGHT WAY

The toothbrush once said to the toilet paper, "I reckon I've got the worst job in the world." The toilet paper replied, "Yah, right!"

The purpose of this chapter is to help you realise that looking after your mouth requires some effort on your part. However, it is not the worst job around. It can be easy and straightforward if done properly. We will be dealing with the various issues in a question and answer format. My hope is to answer any question that might arise.

Why do I need to brush my teeth?

Some people might find this question a bit silly. I have included it because of my experience with a nineteen year old patient who refused to brush her teeth because she claimed she was scared of the whole process. She just couldn't see any reason good enough to make her brush. As you can imagine, the results were disastrous. It is absolutely necessary to clean your mouth to keep it in a healthy state. The bacterial plaque which is mainly responsible for decay and gum disease has constantly to be removed.

How do I brush?

There is no hard and fast rule for brushing. The most important thing is that the technique used should result in a satisfactory reduction of plaque without causing damage to the mouth. The technique I show to my patients is to move your toothbrush in small circular motions as you manoeuvre to different areas of the mouth. It is helpful to be methodical in brushing. This reduces the chance of missing out on some areas.The best way to learn how to brush effectively is to ask your dentist or hygienist to demonsrate to you how to go about it. It is also important to always remember to brush, not scrub.

Where in my mouth should I brush?

You should clean every part of your mouth: teeth, tongue, the roof of your mouth, gums and cheeks. When brushing the teeth, you should aim at cleaning three surfaces: the tongue side, the cheek side and the biting surface. It is also important to pay attention to the neck of the tooth as plaque easily forms here.

How long should I brush for?

Again, there is no rule, but you should brush long enough to get your mouth clean. Some have suggested two minutes (thirty seconds for each quadrant) The more skilled you become the less time you will need, but obviously one second – which is what some of my patients spend – is ridiculous. Spending a minimum time of two minutes is a good guideline to follow. I would also advise you to clean your mouth at least twice a day, in the morning and at night before going to bed.

What are disclosing tablets?

These are tablets which dissolve in water and can be used to expose plaque left over after brushing the teeth. They do this by staining plaque, enabling you to detect areas not properly cleaned.

What toothbrush should I use?

Most toothbrushes are okay, but the one I usually recommend has a small head with medium strength bristles. This design enables you to reach far back into your mouth. Electric toothbrushes are quite common nowadays and can be effective when properly used. People who have problems with movement – who suffer from arthritis, for example – find them particularly useful.

How do I look after my toothbrush and when should I change it?

After brushing your teeth rinse the brush with clean water, making sure that excess toothpaste is removed. Remove the dampness from the brush by shaking it and allow it to dry out before using it again. Your brush is ready to be changed when the bristles start to become flattened. In this state it is less effective and encourages the growth of bacteria.

Which toothpaste should I use?

Which toothpaste to use is a matter of personal preference. Most toothpastes contain fluoride, which provides useful protection against decay. Some types of toothpaste are used to help treat sensitive teeth. It is however important to understand that the most important factor in cleaning your teeth is the mechanical action you perform with your toothbrush.

What is flossing and how do I floss?

Floss is used to clean areas not accessible to normal tooth brushing, for example, between your teeth. It is an important part of dental hygiene. Get about 45 centimeters of dental floss, press it gently against the side of each tooth and move it up and down, as well as back and forth. This will dislodge embedded materials. You can then start on a different tooth with a clean section. Your dentist or hygienist can show you how to use it efficiently. Flossing should be done with care as it can damage the gums if not properly used. Flossing every day is considered okay.

There are also interdental brushes which come in different sizes and can be used to clean between your teeth. Interspatial brushes are also available and are quite useful in cleaning around crowns, bridges and crowded teeth.

Can I use only mouthwash to clean my mouth?

The cleaning of your mouth, and especially your teeth, is achieved mainly by the mechanical action of your toothbrush. There are many types of mouth rinses available. These different types have specific funtions. They include Antiseptic mouthwashes which can be effective against bacteria and can also freshen the breath and Fluoride rinses which can strengthen the teeth and prevent tooth decay. There are also alcohol free mouthwashes that don't give the tingly sensation experienced with those containing alcohol. Your dentist can also prescribe mouthwashes in the treatment of gum disease. It is a good idea to discuss which one to use with your dentist. Mouthwash can be used as an adjunct, but cannot replace tooth brushing.

I bleed from my gums. Should I stop brushing or flossing?

Brushing shouldn't make your gums bleed. If it does, it suggests that your gums are inflamed. This is the time to keep on brushing rather than stop. Brushing should be directed at removing the source of the inflammation, which is usually plaque. You may need to see your dentist or hygienist to discuss this. If there is uncontrolled bleeding in any area of your mouth, you should consult your dentist immediately, as this is not normal.

How do I know I've got bad breath? Can I smell it myself?

It is not easy to detect your own bad breath. Breathing into your hand, as some people suggest, is not a true test because we tend to get used to our own smell. The problem is that even your friend may not tell you for fear of causing offence. You can however ask a family member. Bad breath is a common problem and your dentist will be ready to help you.

What can cause bad breath, apart from poor oral hygiene?

Some kinds of food are notorious for causing bad breath: dairy products, such as milk, cheese, yoghurt, and some spicy foods. Giving your mouth a good clean after eating these would help. It is however recommended that you wait for about an hour after eating before brushing. A common trigger for bad breath is a dry mouth.This may be caused by alcohol, smoking, some medications, infrequent eating or stress.

At what age should I start taking my children to the dentist?

As soon as they start having teeth. A visit also helps them get used to the surroundings. Most dentist don't mind giving them a ride on the chair.

Should I brush my baby's teeth?

Yes you should. There are soft brushes and toothpastes designed for children at each developmental stage. Remember to only use a pea-sized portion of toothpaste, and encourage your child to spit out.

It is good practice to assist your child's tooth brushing up to the age of about seven.

My son plays cricket and wants a mouth guard. Is it necessary?

It is absolutely necessary. A mouth guard is an appliance made to cushion the mouth, teeth and jaw, protecting them from injury. It is usually worn on the upper teeth. It is important to wear a mouth guard when involved in contact sports like cricket, hockey, football, boxing, American football and other activities like cycling, skateboarding and gymnastics.

There are three main types: The ready-made stock mouth guards that you can get in most sporting good stores, the mouth-formed ones that are placed in boiling water and then moulded to the teeth and the custom-made mouth guards that are individually designed and made professionally.

The custom-made ones provide the best fit and are the most comfortable.

Because children are still growing, their mouth guards may need to be replaced regularly to enable proper fitting. It is a good idea to have them checked by your dentist.

Mouth guards are also known to reduce the likelihood of injury to the head, neck and even the brain. Adults who participate in sports should also use them.

It is unwise to sustain an injury when it can be prevented. Use a mouth guard.

What do I do when a tooth is knocked out?

Do not panic. You might be in a position to save someone else's smile.

Look for the tooth and handle the top part only. Do not hold it by the root as this can cause damage to the ligaments. Check if the tooth is clean and put it back into the socket. Hold it in place by biting on a clean handkerchief and get to the dentist as soon as possible.

If you cannot manage to put it back, keep it in the mouth or put it in a cup of milk. This will prevent the tooth from drying out and becoming damaged. If possible do not store in water as the chlorine it contains may damage the roots. Get to the dentist or hospital right away.

It is important to realise that the earlier the tooth is replaced, the better the chance of success.

Why are my teeth stained?

Teeth can either be stained on the outside (surface) or inside (within).

The surface stains are superficial and are usually caused by plaque, food and drinks such as red wine, coffee, tea, curry and some fried foods. Iron tablets, which may cause black stains, smoking and some mouthwashes are other causes.

These stains can be removed by brushing and in some cases by professional cleaning. Some stains however become embedded into the teeth after a long period of contact with them, for example, a lifetime of smoking. A professional clean might not be sufficient to get rid of such stains and your dentist will discuss alternative ways of removing them.

On the other hand, stains that occur on the inside can be due to age. Teeth generally darken with age. It can also be due to tetracycline antibiotics if used in children with developing teeth. This can cause brown and grey stains. Stains on the inside will not rub off. Your dentist will need to assess the stains and decide on the appropriate treatment for you.

As an elderly person, should I expect to lose my teeth?

No. It is possible to keep your teeth for life. Older people do, however, have changes taking place in their mouths, such as gum shrinkage leading to sensitivity.

Also, cleaning your teeth may be a problem if you have difficulty moving your hands. Your dentist will advise you how to get around this. If you are housebound, there are domiciliary services you can contact. And remember, no matter what your age, tooth decay and gum disease can be prevented.

KEY POINTS

- *Looking after your mouth requires some effort on your part. This is easy and straightforward if done properly.*
- *It is possible to keep your teeth for life.*

THE SECRETS

We have now arrived at our promised destination. The secrets have been revealed:

Secret 1: Have a good knowledge of your mouth.
Secret 2: Know the functions of your mouth.
Secret 3: Be aware of changes in your mouth.
Secret 4: Know what to avoid.
Secret 5: Cultivate a healthy eating habit.
Secret 6: Visit your dentist regularly.
Secret 7: Take care of your mouth the right way.

Out of all these, secret 6(visit your dentist regularly) I believe is the corner stone of them all. From the time we first start having teeth we need regular check ups. The same principle applies to keeping your car safely on the road. Any faults will be detected when it goes in for its MOT. A professional can give you expert advice about your mouth. Changes can be monitored and treated if needs be. Sinister problems can be nipped in the bud. The dentist is trained for this and his services should be used. I have observed that most of my patients' problems could have been avoided had they attended regularly. Ask your dentist about the proper technique for brushing. I'm sure there will be no extra charge for this! Most dentists are quite happy to give such advice, or they may refer you to their hygienist who is similarly trained.

Finally, there is no point in having the secret map if you are not going to get the treasure. Now that you know the secrets to having a healthy and attractive mouth, be sure to share them with anyone you feel also needs to know. You can keep your teeth for life, you can have a beautiful smile. The choice is yours.

FINAL WORD

Oral health is such an important part of overall health, it is vital to take good care of your mouth. Apart from making your breath smell better, good oral hygiene will make you feel great.

About the Author

Dr. Ola Lawson has been a general dental practitioner for fourteen years with a special interest in preventive dentistry.

He believes that the toothbrush and toothpaste is incomplete without knowledge.

Fondly known by his patients as the 'friendly dentist', he has successfully motivated a lot of them into achieving a healthy and stable mouth by sharing with them the knowledge required.

Besides working at Cuffley and Stevenage, he runs a domiciliary dental practice for the elderly and disabled.

Ola is married to an actress and blessed with three children.